The Comfortable Breastfeeding Guide

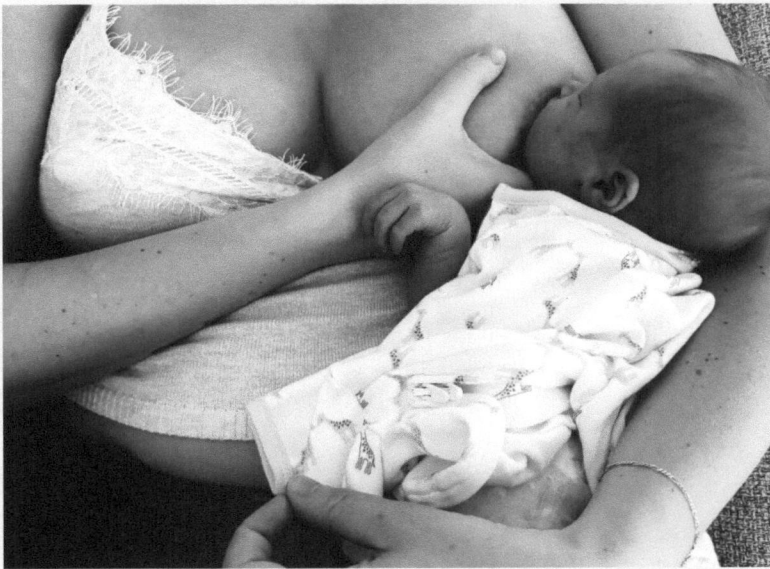

By Kaley Kroschinsky, IBCLC

I0090427

The Comfortable Breastfeeding Guide

By Kaley Kroschinsky, IBCLC

Edited by Andrea Frank-Henkart & Laura Ellie

Photo Credits: Virginia Nymeyer, Laura Ellie, & Kaley Kroschinsky

Copyright First Edition, 2025

This book is dedicated to my Mother, who breastfed me from the moment I left my incubator, and nursed my tiny body back to health.

Also to my own two children, who continue to be my greatest teachers.

And to every Mother who feels the call to breastfeed her baby despite adversity...

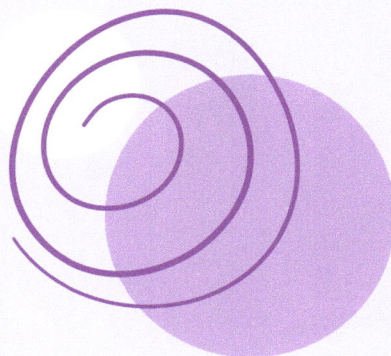

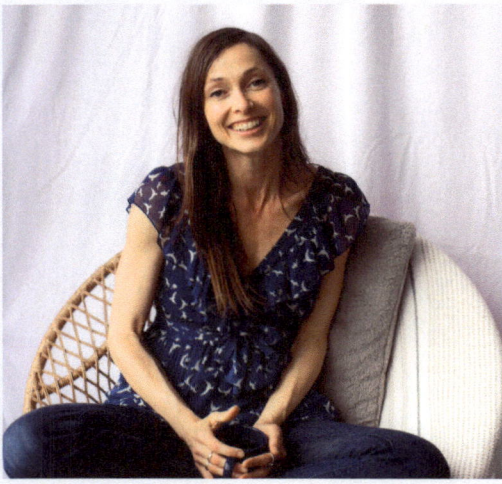

Welcome!

I am so grateful that you have found this resource! This little book contains a wealth of breastfeeding information, tips, and tricks, all accumulated over more than twenty years of working with families, as well 7 years of breastfeeding my own children. Whether you are pregnant and preparing for your first breastfeeding journey, or currently breastfeeding and looking for more help, this guide has something for you.

Your baby's latch is important for many reasons. A shallow latch creates pain and discomfort, which happens to be the number one reason that Mothers give up on breastfeeding. In contrast, when babies are able to latch deeply, breastfeeding feels much more comfortable. Babies with a deep latch are able to drain more milk from your breasts. And when your breasts are well drained, you are able to produce more breastmilk! This is the positive breastfeeding cycle that I want for all of you!

But before you read on, I want to acknowledge that breastfeeding is natural, but that certainly doesn't mean that it's easy. Many routine birth and postpartum procedures interfere with the establishment of early breastfeeding, leaving Mothers wondering where things went wrong. (See the final section of this book, for a Postpartum & Infant Feeding Preferences guide, that will help you to prioritize early breastfeeding). The reality is that not all babies will latch, and not all Moms will produce a full supply of breastmilk. But too often, Moms feel alone in their breastfeeding struggles, or like something is wrong with them. In contrast, when families are able to access good information and support from the start, they are a lot more likely to feel empowered in their feeding experiences. I believe that we were never meant to do this alone, and by reading this book, you are giving yourself a wealth of information and tools. However, this book was not intended to replace the support of a qualified Lactation Consultant, breastfeeding counsellor and/or group of breastfeeding Moms. Please connect if you are having trouble finding lactation support in your local area!

My Own Early Breastfeeding Challenges

My first son was what is sometimes referred to in the lactation world as a " barracuda". In other words, he was a voracious breastfeeder with a suck to rip your fingernails off. His intense suck and ravenous appetite created an avalanche of troubles for us.

First of all, I had to watch my baby's latch like a hawk. One false move and my nipples would become cracked, bloody and very sore. Thanks to my midwifery background and attention to detail, I was able to avoid major nipple damage... But it wasn't the bonding experience I had hoped for. Second, my supply responded to the aggressive stimulation, and we were both swimming in breastmilk. My oversupply led to frequent clogged ducts. Meanwhile my son became gassy and uncomfortable, and was spitting up large volumes of milk after every feed. It was messy and sad to see my baby uncomfortable so often.

Thankfully after a month of struggling, I attended a local breastfeeding circle where I learned about laid back breastfeeding, and it changed everything for us!

Laid Back Breastfeeding & How Everything Changed.

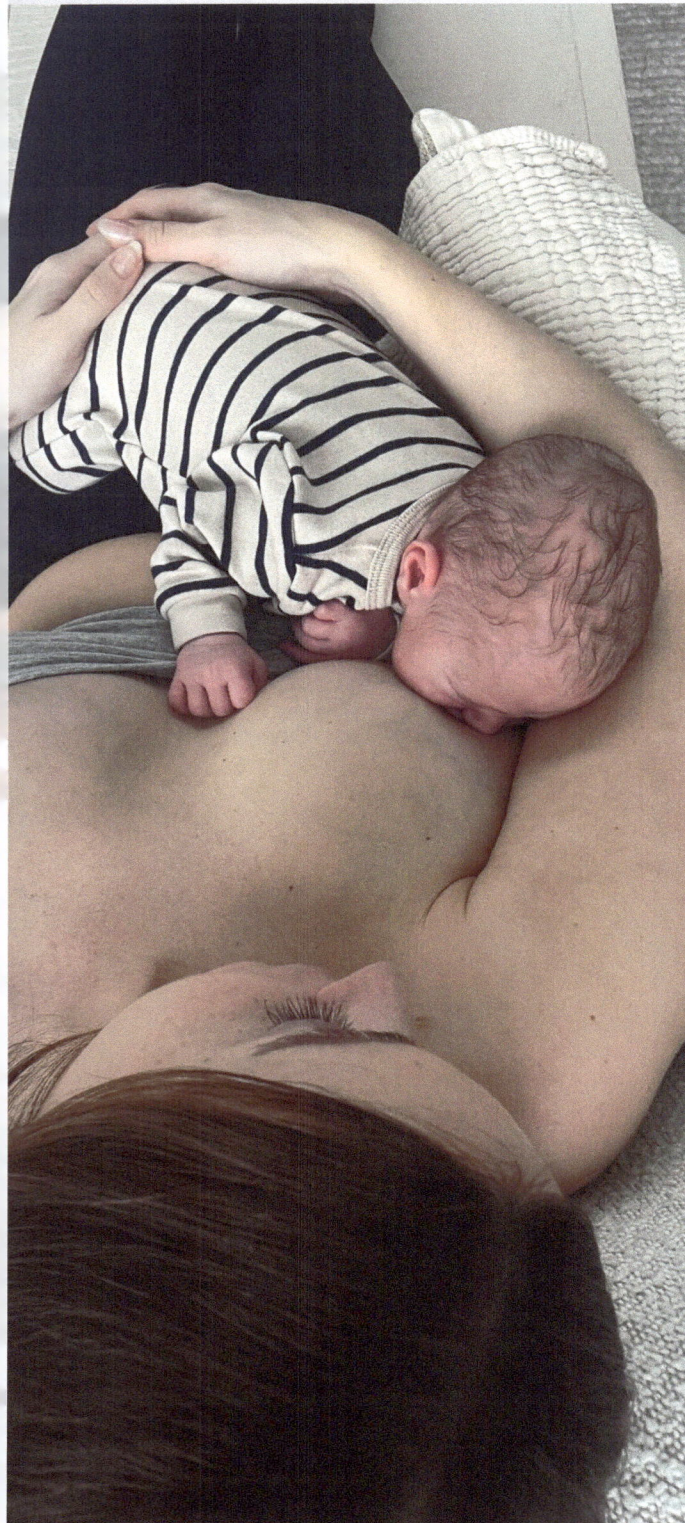

The simple act of laying back to breastfeed gave my baby the ability to manage the flow of my milk, and he became a happy baby! Breastfeeding became more comfortable and I didn't have to watch carefully with every latch. My baby stopped spitting up excessively, which made it easier to leave the house. But more importantly, I started to fall in love with breastfeeding.

How was all of this possible with a simple position change? What I learned was that laid back or Natural Breastfeeding Positions (also known as Biological Nurturing), stimulate a baby's inborn breastfeeding instincts. A deeper latch is achieved thanks to gravity, as well as the way a baby's primitive neonatal reflexes are stimulated when they are on top of you doing the breast crawl.

Natural Breastfeeding Positions set up the ideal training ground for early breastfeeding. A deeper latch is a more comfortable latch, and results in better milk transfer. Babies are born with the natural ability to latch and breastfeed themselves. We just have to give them the chance!

Breastfeeding Is Not The Same As Formula Feeding.

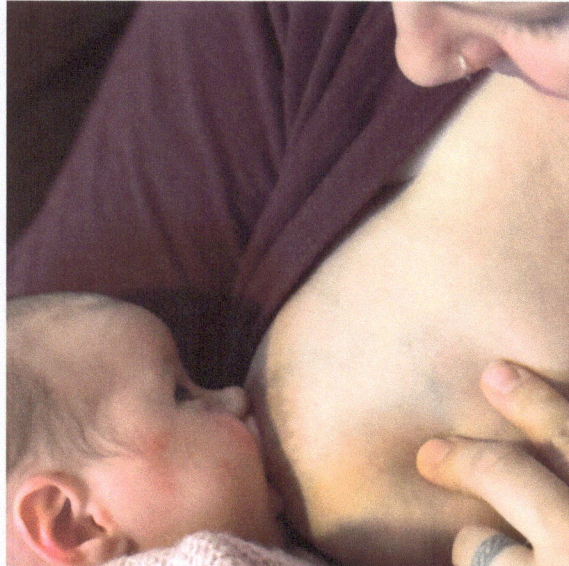

The thing that really surprised me, was that I had been a midwife for 5 years before having my first baby. I had participated in a breastfeeding education course during my Midwifery training, and I had helped countless women latch and breastfeed their babies for the first time. How did I not know about this life-changing breastfeeding method?

What I realized was that like many healthcare professionals, I had been trained to treat breastfeeding more like formula feeding. After a few generations of formula feeding dominance in North America, our culture has become more familiar with bottles and formula, than with the natural act of breastfeeding. And as a healthcare professional, I was trained to teach women to breastfeed in a way that mimicked bottle feeding. But these methods don't work for many women, and they didn't work for me. The reality is that over 80% of first time mothers report significant breastfeeding difficulties within the first week. Something isn't working about the way that most women are being taught to breastfeed their babies. Breastfeeding is as much art as it is science, and when Mothers are taught to view breastfeeding in an overly mechanistic way, they miss out on some pieces that can ultimately make breastfeeding easier, more comfortable and more enjoyable.

The Breast Crawl: We are Mammals!

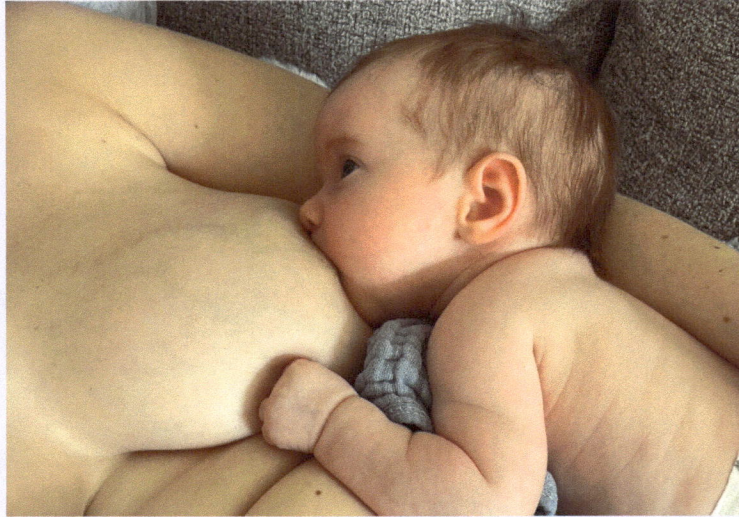

One false belief in our culture is that babies are completely helpless when they are born. This is why many people are amazed to learn about "The Breast Crawl", or the innate ability for newborns to crawl and latch themselves after birth. Like other mammals, human babies are capable of crawling to the breast and latching themselves! The best time to start the breast crawl and to utilize laid-back breastfeeding, is immediately after birth. But don't worry if you miss the immediate postpartum window; you can always recreate this process during your baby's first days and weeks!

To set up the breast crawl, start by placing your baby skin to skin, with their tummy on top of your tummy, just below one of your breasts. Your baby's reflexes will be stimulated, and they may start bobbing their head and/or making crawling movements with their arms and legs. It may take your baby some time to become familiar with your body. Baby's hands may touch and massage your breast, and they may mouth and lick at your nipple. They may even let out a little cry. Gently hold and shape your breast just behind your areola, to help your baby to find their way. After some time and patience, your baby will latch themselves. Try to keep still at first, as your baby settles in. Eventually, your baby will begin to suckle! If your baby wiggles up too high and misses your nipple, gently bring them back down to your tummy and try again. This can all happen within the first hour or two after birth. If you were given medications during labour, or if your baby is preterm, their reflexes may not be as strong at first.

Where Do I Start?

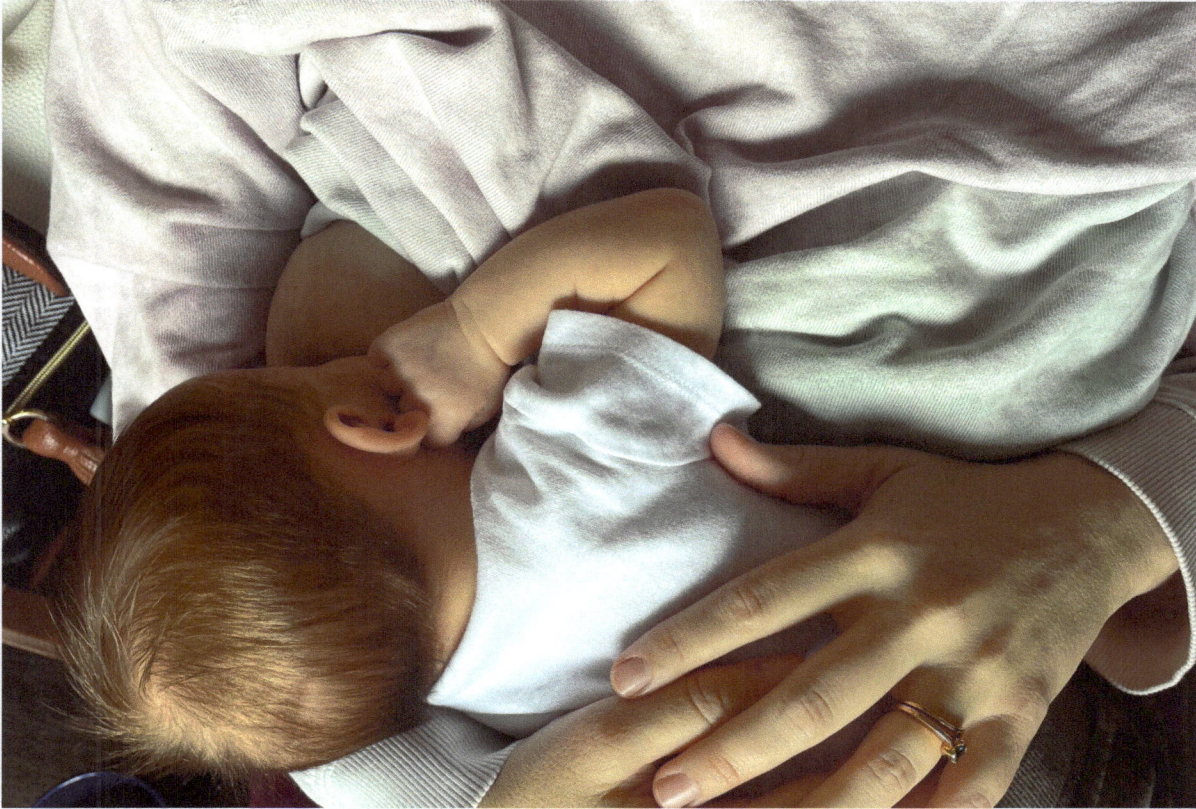

1) **If you are currently pregnant** and preparing to breastfeed, we recommend starting with the breast crawl (as described on the previous page). The breast crawl brings you and your baby into a Natural Breastfeeding Position, which is an ideal position for learning and reinforcing a deep latch. Laid back breastfeeding positions are also more comfortable for your breasts, nipples, and for your body in general. Please see our "Early Postpartum and Infant Feeding Preferences" guide, which can help to serve as a roadmap for early breastfeeding.

2) **If you are currently breastfeeding** and struggling with nipple pain and/or damage, a shallow latch is the prime suspect. There are other culprits, which we will get into later. But no matter what, *having a deep latch is essential to your breastfeeding comfort and success*. Laid-back breastfeeding positions take advantage of gravity as well as your baby's inborn breastfeeding instincts, to create the deepest latch possible. These positions make breastfeeding more comfortable, so that you can relax and enjoy feeding your baby!

How To Practice Laid Back Breastfeeding

A) **GET COMFORTABLE**

Find a place where you can lie back enough to rest your head. Use extra pillows to support your arms, so that you can relax your shoulders away from your ears.

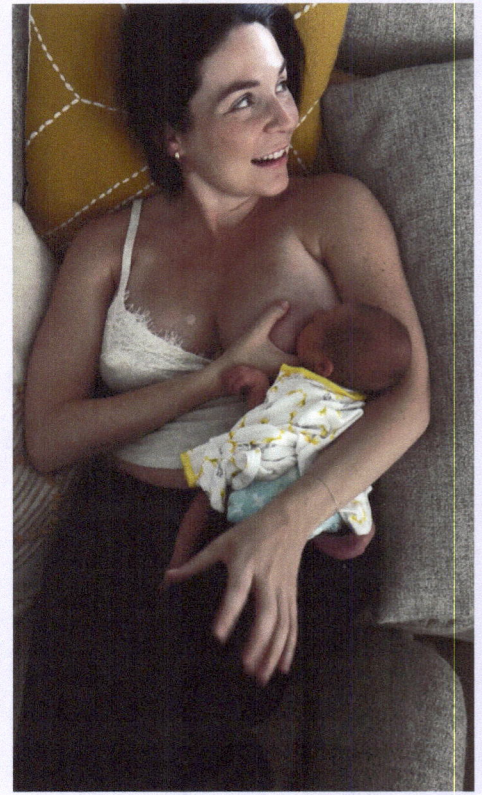

B) **USE GRAVITY TO CONNECT YOUR BABY'S BODY TO YOURS**

Bring your baby tummy to tummy, using gravity to anchor their body onto yours. Decide which side they are going to feed on, then use that same arm like a pillow to keep your baby from falling to one side. Place your baby with their chin below your areola, so that they have to look up towards the tip of your nipple.

C) **SHAPE YOUR BREAST, & ENCOURAGE YOUR BABY TO LATCH DEEPLY WHILE AIMING THE TIP OF YOUR NIPPLE TO THE ROOF OF YOUR BABY'S MOUTH**

Use your opposite hand to gently shape your breast just behind your areola, so that your baby can get a big mouthful. Allow your baby to bob around and let them find your nipple, without moving your breast to your baby. Keep shaping your breast for the first part of the latch, and try to get as much breast tissue into your baby's mouth as possible. Your baby's chin will be the anchor for their latch, and there should be some space for their nose.

D) **ADJUST AS NEEDED TO MAKE IT COMFORTABLE**

If your baby has latched to only the tip of your nipple, or if the latch is painful, unlatch by sliding your finger into the corner of your baby's mouth to break the seal. The deeper the latch, the more comfortable it will feel, and the less your nipples will become damaged... So be patient, and try for a deep latch with every feed.

Extra Tips When Using
Laid Back Breastfeeding

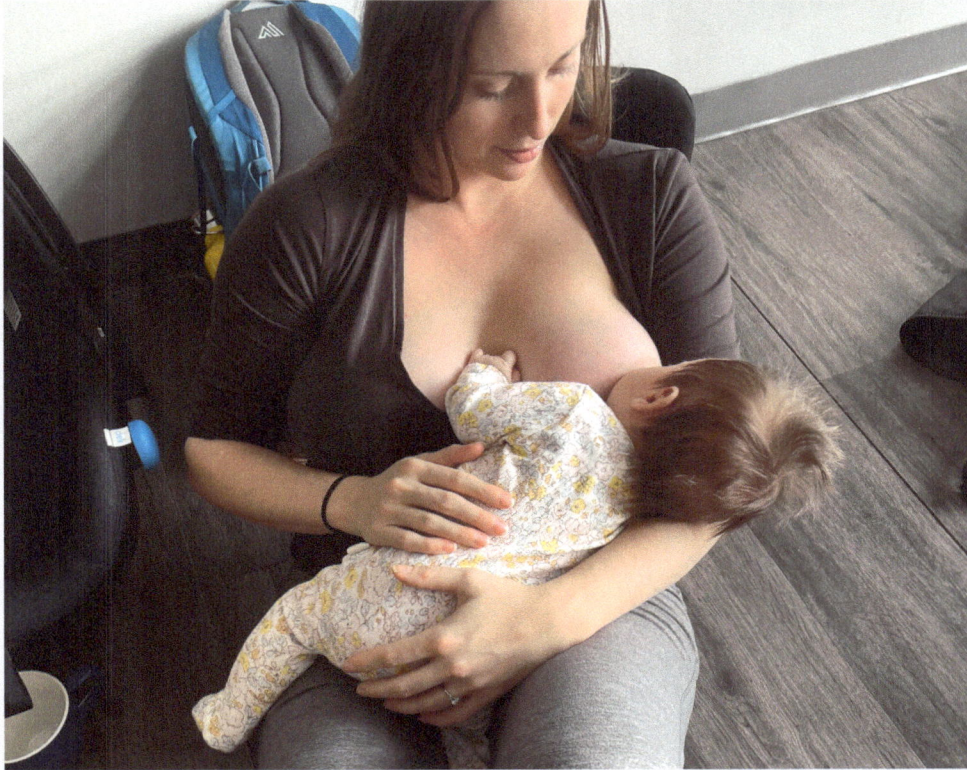

- Your positioning will somewhat depend on your breast size. Moms with larger breasts will usually have to recline further. *Position your baby where your breast naturally falls, rather than moving your breast to your baby.*

- If your baby is struggling to latch in a laid back position, try this trick. Latch first in a familiar position like an upright cradle position, then recline back once your baby has latched. This will require you to "scoot" your hips forward, so that baby can come to rest on top of you. Make sure that your baby is completely "tummy to tummy", and that you feel comfortable.

- Try practicing laid back positions in the bath! Bathing with your baby can be a restful and comfortable way to practice breastfeeding.

- Allow your baby to straddle one of your legs while feeding, as a way to connect them and give them foot contact.

Establishing A Deep Latch:

An important point to reiterate is that your baby's chin is the anchor of their latch. To establish a deep latch, think about bringing your baby's chin to your breast, (rather than their nose), which will stimulate their mouth to open wide. Aim the tip of your nipple towards the roof of your baby's mouth, and as they open their mouth, allow them to take in as much of your nipple, areola and breast tissue as possible. The tip of your nipple must be at your baby's soft palate towards the back of their mouth, for the latch to be comfortable. If the latch is painful, you can always unlatch and try again. (Break the suction/seal by slipping your finger into the corner of your baby's mouth, and pulling out gently on their cheek.) Your baby should be positioned low enough that they have to look up towards your breast..This will also give them more space to breathe easily through their nose.

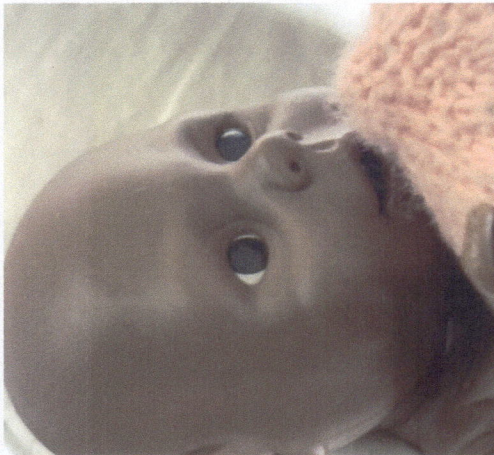

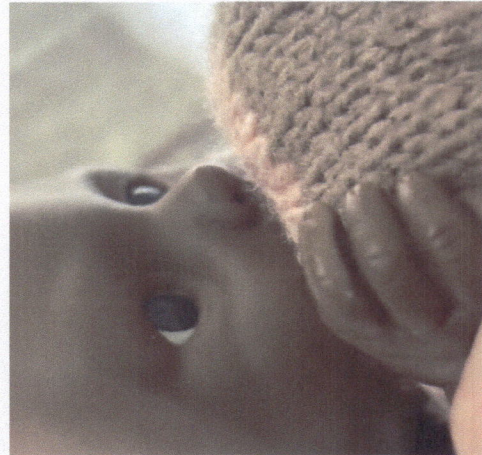

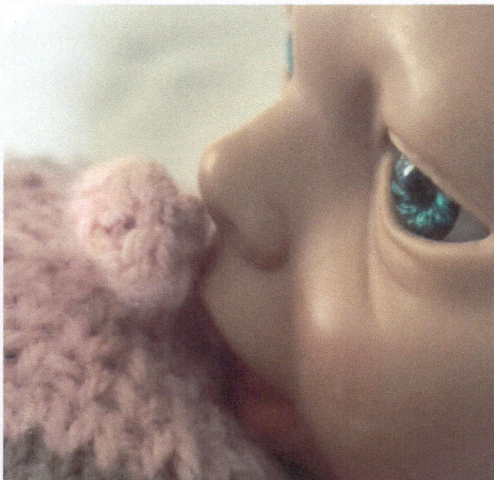

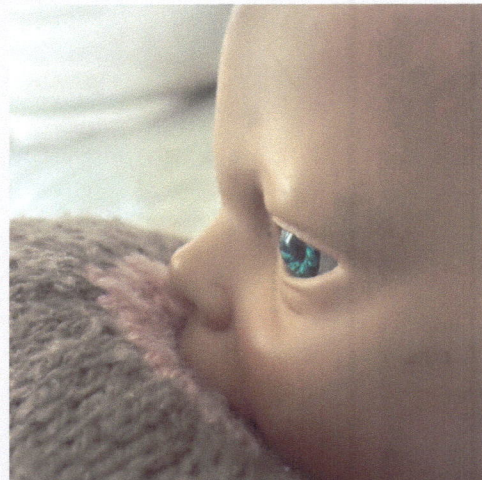

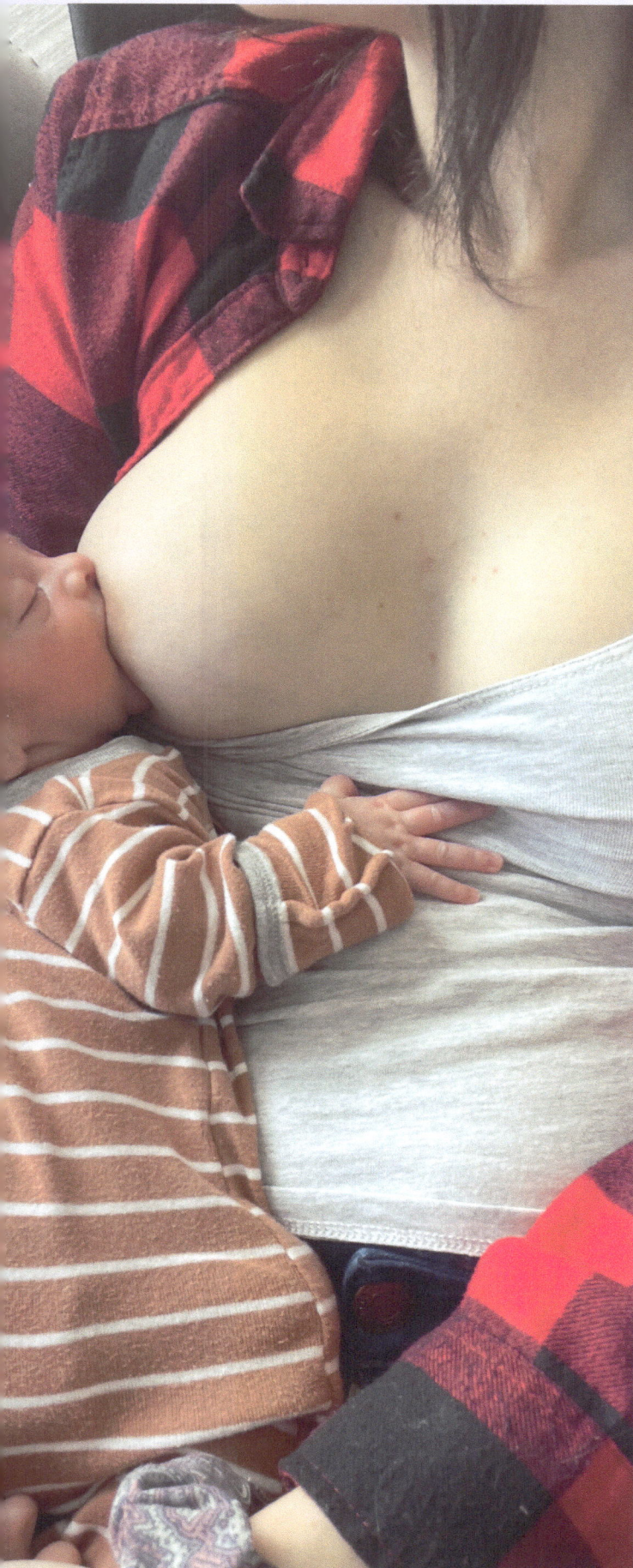

Self Checklist For Laid Back Breastfeeding

✔ No gaps between your body & baby's body.

✔ If you take your hands away for a moment, gravity keeps your baby anchored in place.

✔ Baby's chin is firmly connected to your breast, and their nose is free.

✔ Baby is looking up towards your breast, not tucking their chin.

✔ Baby's feet are anchored.

✔ You feel comfortable, and you have support for your arms and head as needed.

✔ The top & bottom lips are turned out to form a suction, to keep your baby latched.

✔ The latch is as deep as possible, with your nipple aimed at the roof of your baby's mouth.

Other Sources Of Pain...

If you take one thing away from this guide, I hope it is this: ***If you are having challenges with breastfeeding, it is not your fault and there is nothing wrong with you. Breastfeeding is natural, but it doesn't come easily to many Mothers.*** I believe that Mothers were never meant to breastfeed alone. If you practice the techniques in this guide and you are still having trouble, please reach out for support. You can always reach out to us for home, clinic or virtual Lactation support. Or please check your local area for Lactation Consultants, breastfeeding specialists, and/or breastfeeding support groups. **In summary, please don't struggle alone!**

Some breastfeeding challenges will require specialized support, and I don't recommend trying to manage them on your own. Here are some other main offenders of breast/nipple pain.

- Tension in your baby's head, neck, mouth, back: *Sometimes a result of the birth process or pregnancy positioning, these babies often benefit from bodywork, including: Physiotherapy, Osteopathy, Cranio-Sacral Therapy and/or Chiropractic that specialize in infant care.*

- Tongue/oral ties: *When the frenulum under the tongue and/or upper lip causes restrictions, leading to abnormal suck patterns and/or compensations. Oral ties inhibit breastfeeding in around 5% of babies, or maybe more. Many Mothers experience less breastfeeding pain after a procedure to release the tethered tissue, which can help babies to latch more deeply. Babies with oral ties benefit from bodywork (as described above), as well as in-person Lactation support.*

- Mastitis: *Painful swelling within in the breast(s), sometimes caused by a bacterial infection. Mothers usually notice a hard, red, and potentially hot lump that continues to get worse over time. They may feel exhausted or unwell. Please contact your healthcare provider if you think you have mastitis.*

- Nipple Dysbiosis (formerly known as thrush): *An imbalance of yeast/bacteria on the nipple. Mothers will notice sharp, stabbing pain in their breasts and nipples, even between feeds. The baby may show symptoms as well. Contact your healthcare provider or local Lactation Consultant for more information and support!*

- Pumping Trauma: *Beware of pumping with the wrong flange size, pumping for too long, pumping with your suction turned up too high, frequent use of silicone pumps, etc. Ineffective pumping can lead to unexplained pain while breastfeeding, so please reach out to a Lactation Consultant for pumping support, if you think this might be you...*

Congratulations on being proactive, giving yourself the opportunity to learn, and for trying a less conventional approach! I sincerely hope that you have gained some valuable information from this book. Or at the very least, that you feel ready to get comfortable and snuggle up while feeding your baby.

Please connect if you would like to learn more from The MotherTree Collective, or if you would like to participate in any of our classes, circles or meet-ups. If this information has impacted your breastfeeding journey, please let us know. We absolutely love hearing from Mammas & their little ones! With many warm wishes for your breastfeeding adventures,

Kaley Kroschinsky

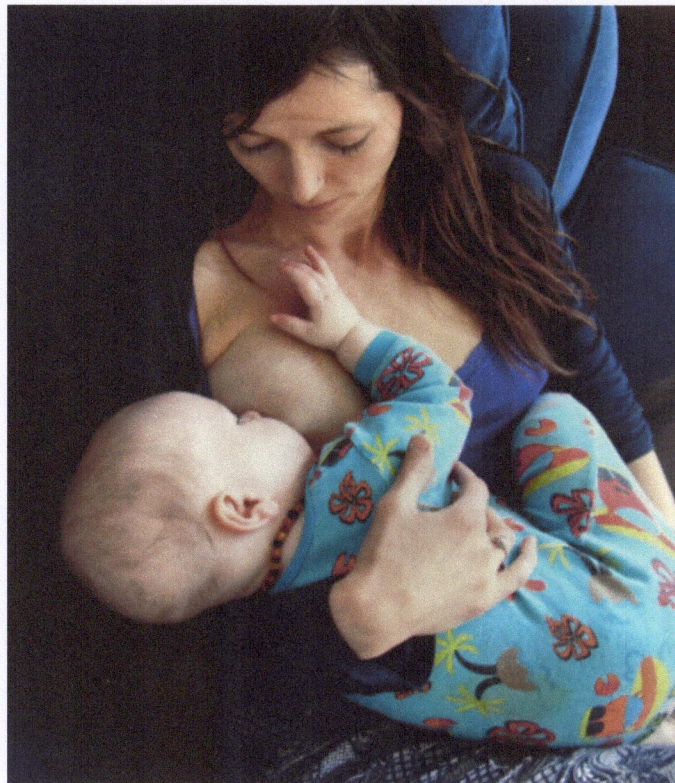

themothertree.ca
kaleykroschinsky@gmail.com
@themothertreecollective

Sources

1) Breimer, Yael. "Lie Back abd Relax! A Look at Laid Back Breastfeeding" (2017). lllusa.org/lie-back-and-relax https://lllusa.org/lie-back-and-relax-a-look-at-laid-back-breastfeeding/

2) Colson, S. The Laid-back Breastfeeding Revolution". http://www.midwiferytoday.com/articles/BiologicalNurturing.

3) Colson, S & Colson J. (2022). Biological Nurturing: "Sample of Biological Nurturing". https://www.biologicalnurturing.com/sample-of-biological-nurturing/ "Biological Nurturing:

4) La Leche League Canada. (August, 2022). *"The First Hours After Birth - The Nine Instinctive Stages".* https://www.lllc.ca/first-hours-after-birth-nine-instinctive-stages

5) La Leche League Canada. (August, 2022). *"The First Hours After Birth - The Nine Instinctive Stages".* https://www.lllc.ca/first-hours-after-birth-nine-instinctive-stages

6) Lingling H, Fan C, et. al. Efficacy of Breast Crawling on Breastfeeding Outcomes, Knowledge, Attitudes, and Anxiety Status After Term Vaginal Birth: A Randomized Controlled Trial. Matern Child Nutr. 2025 Jul 7:e70063. doi: 10.1111/mcn.70063. Epub ahead of print. PMID: 40619948.

7) Milinco M, Travan L, et al. BN (Biological Nurturing) Investigators. Effectiveness of biological nurturing on early breastfeeding problems: a randomized controlled trial. Int Breastfeed J. 2020 Apr 5;15(1):21. doi: 10.1186/s13006-020-00261-4. PMID: 32248838; PMCID: PMC7132959.

8) Mohrbacher, Nancy (2020). *"The Study I've Waited For Is Finally Here".* https://nancymohrbacher.com/blogs/news/the-study-ive-waited-for-is-finally-here

9) Nesbitt, T & Mohrbacher, N. (2024). *"Natural Breastfeeding for an Easier Start".* https://www.naturalbreastfeeding.com/

10) Perinatal Services BC: Birth Preferences Guide: chrome-extension://bdfcnmeidppjeaggnmidamkiddifkdib/viewer.html?file=http://www.perinatalservicesbc.ca/Documents/Health-info/PSBC_Birth_Preference_Guide.pdf

Resource 1:
Early Postpartum & Infant Feeding Preferences.

A guide to support you in your early breastfeeding journey, by listing some of the choices that you may encounter with your newborn. Print a copy to go along with your birth plan, and share with your care providers. This tool can help you to feel informed and empowered in your early postpartum choices, and support you in prioritizing early breastfeeding and/or milk removal.

Resource 2:
Infant Feeding & Output Record

An optional tracking sheet to support you with early breastfeeding. Not everyone needs to track every feed. But it can be helpful for families who are having difficulty, to look for trends, and in communicating with care providers. Print copies of this record to keep beside your bed, and jot down notes as you feed throughout the day.

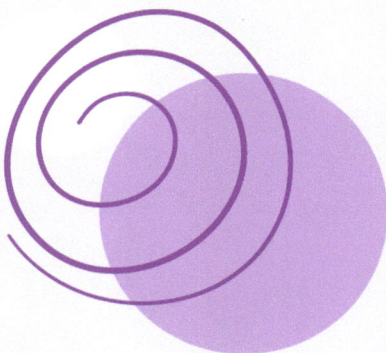

Early Postpartum & Infant Feeding Preferences:

Introduction

Names(s):

Preferred name(s):

Estimated Due Date:
Planned Birth Place:
Birth Team: (Midwives, Physicians, OB, Paediatrician, Doula, etc):

-

-

Background

Thank you for being a part of my baby's birth day! I am grateful that you are taking the time to read my postpartum and infant feeding preferences. These are some things that I would like you to know: (i.e. previous breastfeeding experiences, communication preferences, religious or spiritual beliefs, specific concerns, & anything that you may want extra support with, etc).

-

-

-

Immediate Postpartum

○ Please place my baby skin to skin immediately after the birth, and leave them with me until after their first feed if possible.

○ I would prefer to delay clamping of the umbilical cord if possible.

○ Please give me or my partner the option to cut the umbilical cord if possible.

○ I would prefer space and time for my baby to attempt the breast crawl, and to do our first feed in a reclined position if it feels right.

○ If I have a cesarean birth, I would prefer to do skin to skin contact in the operating room if possible.

○ Please assist me as much as possible with early feeding.

○ Please delay the weight and any newborn procedures, until after the first feed if possible.

○ If my baby and I are separated after the birth, please give my partner the option to do skin to skin with our baby if possible.

○ I have hand expressed my own colostrum, and I would prefer to give my colostrum if my baby requires any supplementation.

○ If there is a delay in early feeding for some reason, please help me to hand express colostrum and/or start pumping right away.

Early Postpartum & Infant Feeding Preferences:

○ I would like to have as much skin to skin contact with my baby as possible.

○ I would prefer to feed my baby on demand, or whenever they are showing feeding cues.

○ I would appreciate as much help as possible with early positions and latch.

○ I have hand expressed some colostrum, and I would prefer to give this first if my baby requires supplementation.

○ I would prefer to use donor milk if my baby requires additional supplementation.

○ Please do not give my baby a pacifier or bottle, unless I have otherwise agreed.

○ If my baby requires supplementation, I would prefer to try syringe or cup feeding before a bottle.

○ If my baby is unable to feed directly from my breast for any reason, please help me with hand expression and/or pumping.

○ Please keep me as informed and involved in my baby's care as possible.

○ Please help me to have as much skin to skin contact as possible during my baby's NICU stay, knowing that this promotes regulation, attachment and feeding.

○ My partner would like to do as much skin to skin as possible.

○ Please help me to start pumping early, and to create a pumping schedule similar to my baby's feeding schedule.

○ Please help me to pump beside my baby, knowing that this supports let down and can increase milk volume.

Newborn Feeding & Output Record

Mom's Name:

(Sample)

Date:

TIME OF FEED	LENGTH OF FEED	RIGHT/ LEFT BOTH SIDES	POSITION	PAIN? 1:10	VOID/BM?	OTHER NOTE
06:25	20/10	R/L	SIDE-LYING	3:10 4:10	V/BM	2ND SIDE 30 M LATER
08:45	25	L ONLY	LAID BACK	2:10	V	LONG NAP
11:45	20/20	R/L	X-CRADLE	3:10 4:10	V/BM	
14:00	15	L	X-CRADLE	4:10	V/BM	LONG NAP
16:45	15/15	R/L	LAID BACK	1:10 2:10	V/BM	
18:00	10	R	X-CRADLE	3:10	V	FUSSY & GAS
19:30	15	L	CARRIER	4:10	V	FUSSY& GASSY
20:45	10	R	X-CRADLE	3:10	BM	LARGE BM
21:30	15/15	L/R	LAID-BACK	2:10 1:10		BED TIME
0015	20	R	SIDE-LYING	2:10	V/BM	BACK TO SLEEP
0300	20	L	SIDE-LYING	3:10	V	CO SLEEP
0500	30	R	SIDE-LYING	2:10	V	CO SLEEP

ewborn Feeding & Output Record

o Print)

Mom's Name:

Date:

TIME OF FEED	LENGTH OF FEED	RIGHT/ LEFT/ BOTH SIDES?	POSITION	PAIN? 1:10	VOID/ BM?	OTHER NOTES